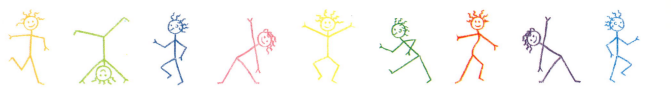

Healthy Eating

By Paul Bennett

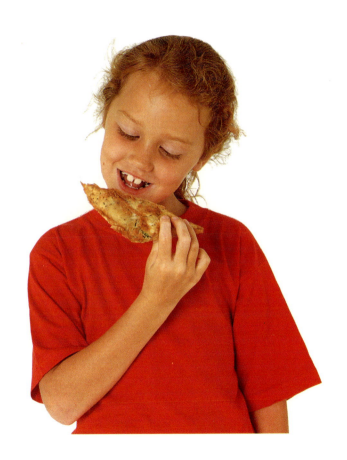

Silver Press
Parsippany, New Jersey

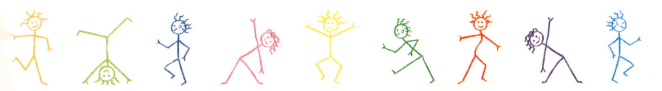

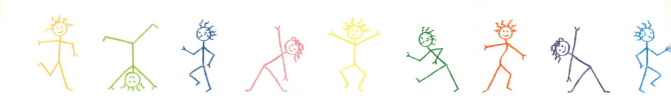

First published in Great Britain in 1997 by

Belitha Press Limited
London House, Great Eastern Wharf
Parkgate Road, London SW11 4NQ

Copyright in this format © Belitha Press Limited 1997
Text copyright © Paul Bennett

Editor: Veronica Ross
Series designer: Hayley Cove
Photographer: Claire Paxton
Illustrator: Cilla Eurich
Picture researcher: Diana Morris
Consultant: Elizabeth Atkinson

All rights reserved, including the right of reproduction,
in whole, or in part, in any form.

Published in the United States in 1998 by

Silver Press
A Division of Simon & Schuster
299 Jefferson Road
Parsippany, New Jersey 07054-0480

Library of Congress Cataloging-in-Publication Data
Bennett, Paul, 1954-
Healthy eating/by Paul Bennett.
Originally published: London: Belitha Press, 1997.
Includes index.
Summary: Discusses healthy eating, including why we need to eat, how to keep a balanced diet, facts about vitamins and minerals, how the digestive system works, and what to do when you eat too much.
1. Nutrition–Juvenile literature. [1. Nutrition.] I. Title. II. Series: Bodyworks (Parsippany, N.J.)
QP141.B515   1998   96-36127
613.2.–dc21   CIP   AC
ISBN 0-382-39779-7 (LSB)   10 9 8 7 6 5 4 3 2 1
ISBN 0-382-39780-0 (PBK)   10 9 8 7 6 5 4 3 2 1

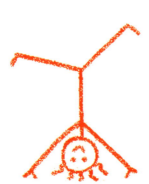

Printed in Hong Kong

Photo credits
Axiom/Jim Holmes: 27t. Zefa/Stockmarket/Craig Tuttle: 17t.

Thanks to models Meera, Jodie, Sam, Topel, Ricky

Words in **bold** are explained in the list
of useful words on pages 30 and 31.

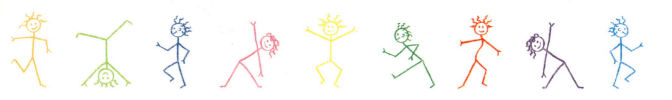

Contents

Why do I need to eat?	4
A balanced diet	6
Body-building foods	8
Energy foods	10
Fatty foods	12
Vitamins and minerals	14
All about fiber	16
Water for life	18
Chewing and swallowing	20
Digesting your food	22
Snacks and junk food	24
Special food	26
I ate too much!	28
Useful words	30
Index	32

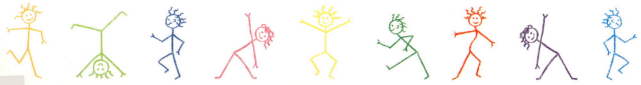

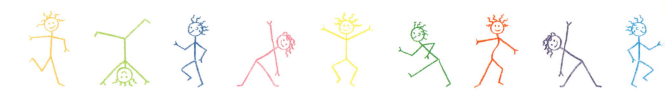

Why do I need to eat?

Food keeps you alive. You need to eat in order to stay **healthy** and feel fit and well.

The useful parts of food, called **nutrients**, are used to help your body grow and **repair** itself.

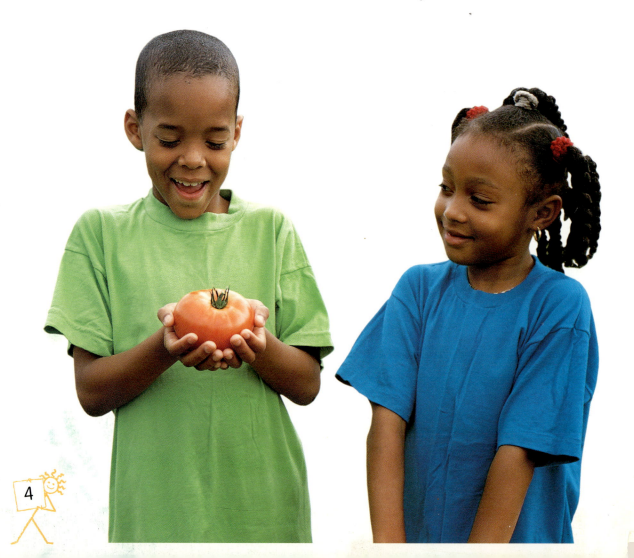

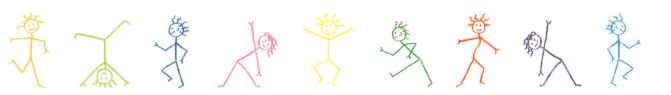

Food is body fuel. It gives you **energy** for playing and working. Your body uses energy all the time.

It is important to eat three meals every day to stay healthy and feel good.

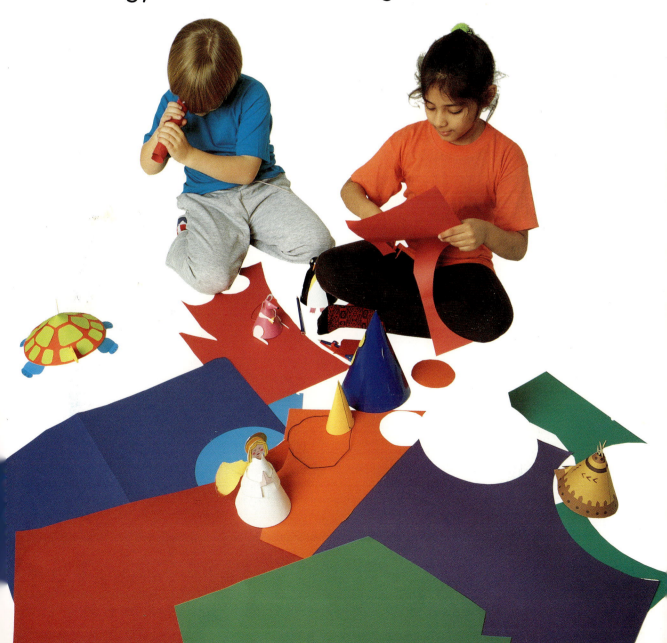

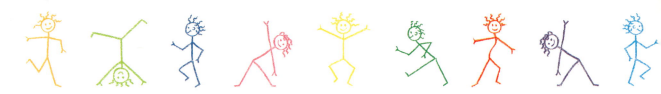

A balanced diet

There are lots of different types of food. Fruit, meat, vegetables, bread, and cheese are just a few.

Can you think of any more?

What are your favorite foods?

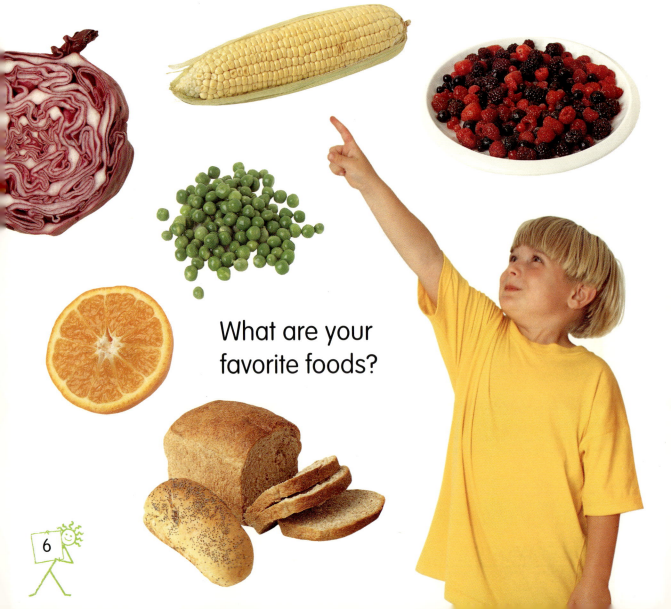

The food you eat every day is called your diet. A balanced diet is one that has all the nutrients your body needs.

Different foods have different nutrients in them. To stay healthy, you need to eat different types of food so that you get all the nutrients you need.

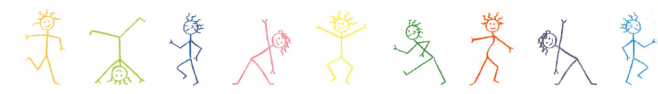

Body-building foods

Body-building foods are rich in **proteins**. Proteins build your **muscles**, skin, **bones**, and all the other parts of your body.

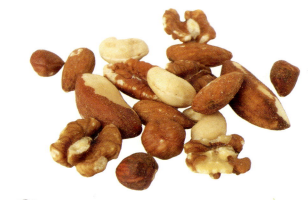

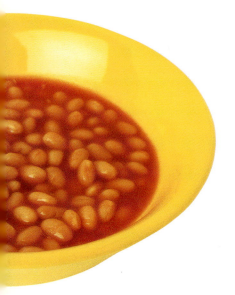

Proteins help you grow. They also help your body repair itself.

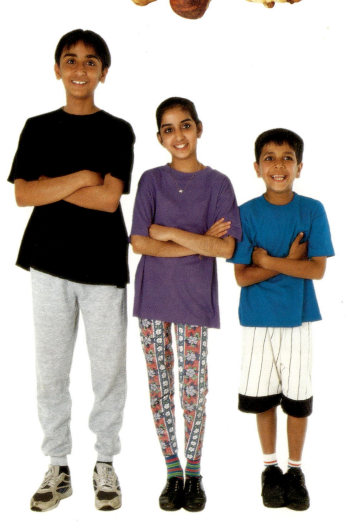

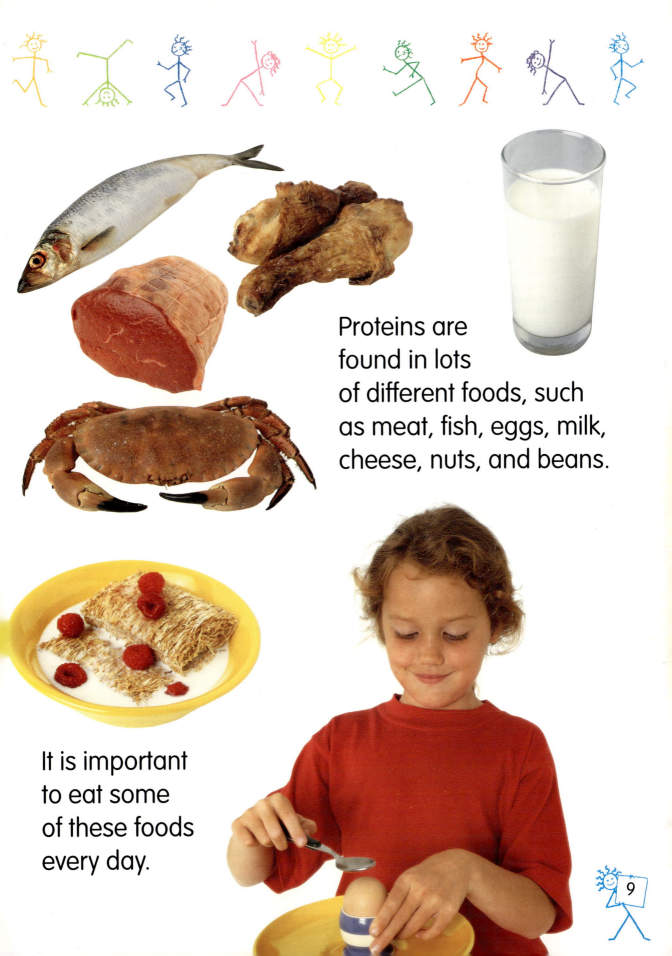

Proteins are found in lots of different foods, such as meat, fish, eggs, milk, cheese, nuts, and beans.

It is important to eat some of these foods every day.

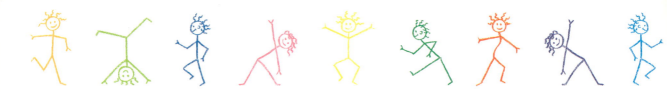

Energy foods

You use up lots of energy when you are running around. Energy comes from foods that are rich in **carbohydrates**.

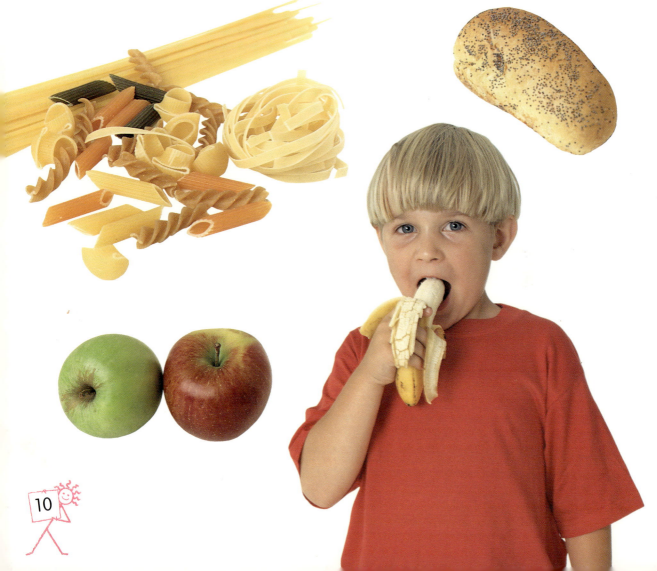

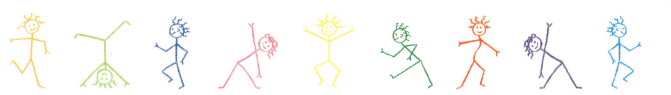

Carbohydrates are found in potatoes, rice, pasta, bread, and fruit.

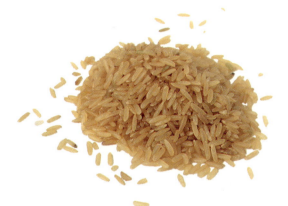

You need lots of these foods if you are exercising or playing games.

Sweet foods, such as cake and chocolate, are full of carbohydrates too. But too much cake and chocolate can make you unhealthy.

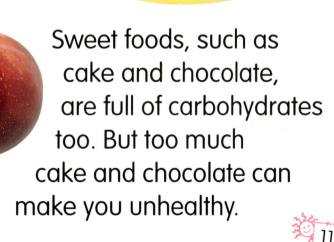

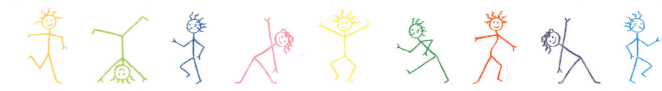

Fatty foods

You only need a small amount of fat in your diet to stay healthy.

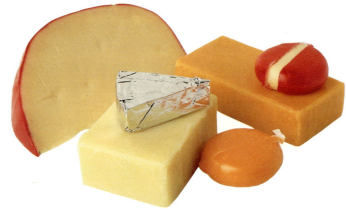

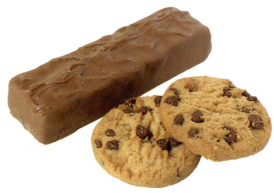

Fats are found in foods such as butter, cheese, chocolate, and cookies.

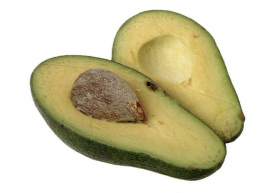

Avocados, vegetable oils, sardines, and meat also contain lots of fat.

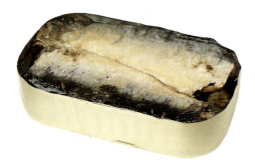

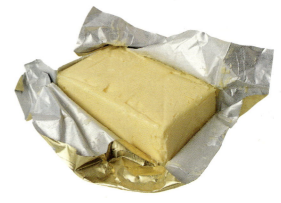

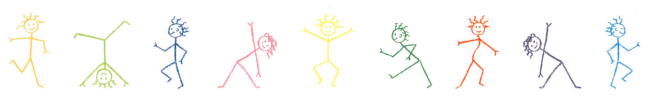

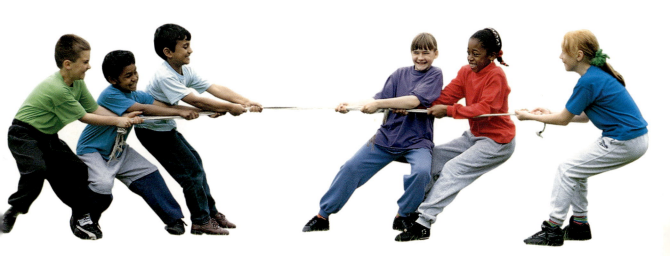

Many people try to cut down the amount of fat in their diet. They grill food instead of frying it, and they use skimmed milk (milk without the cream).

If you eat too many fatty foods, such as these fried **samosas**, you may become overweight.

Fats give you lots of energy.

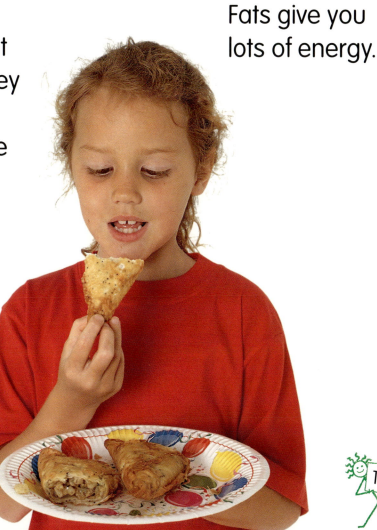

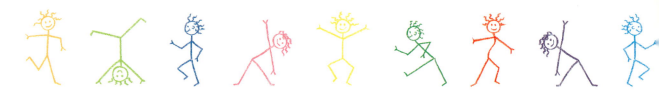

Vitamins and minerals

A balanced diet will give you all the **vitamins** and **minerals** you need.

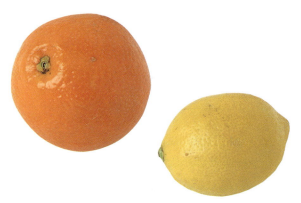

There are many different kinds of vitamins. They keep your body working properly.

Vitamin C is found in vegetables and fruit. It helps cuts heal, and helps you fight off colds and flu.

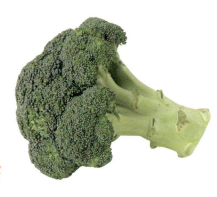

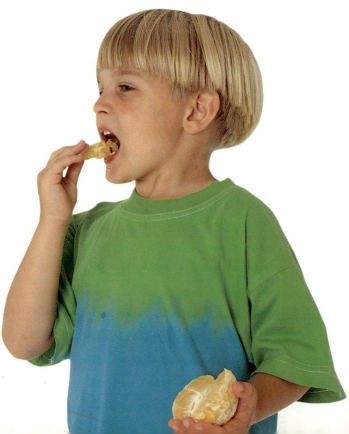

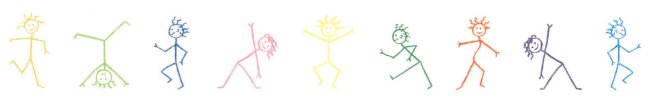

Vitamins and minerals are found in many different foods. Fish, oranges, and tomatoes contain vitamins.

Milk, cheese, and green vegetables are good sources of minerals.

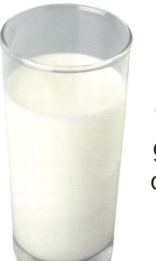

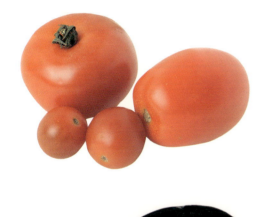

Calcium is a mineral found in milk. It helps keep your bones and teeth healthy and strong.

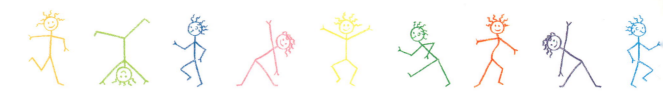

All about fiber

Fiber is an important part of a balanced diet. It does not have any nutrients, but it helps you **digest** the food you eat.

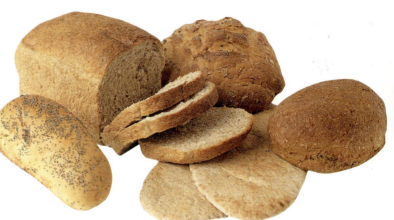

Fiber also helps fill you up.

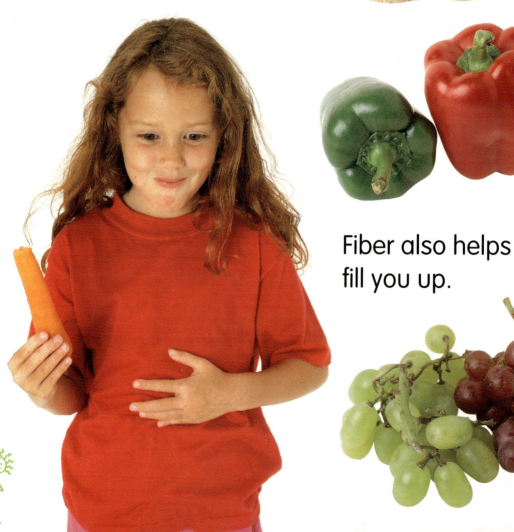

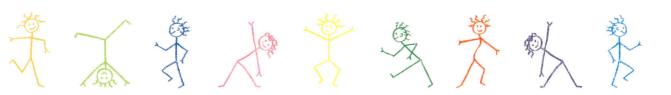

Fiber is found in plants like the wheat shown here. Flour is made from wheat. It is used to make bread.

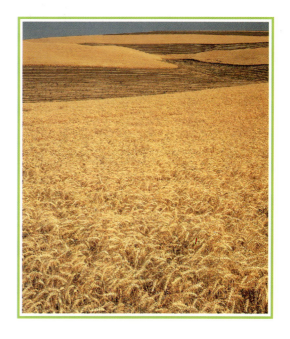

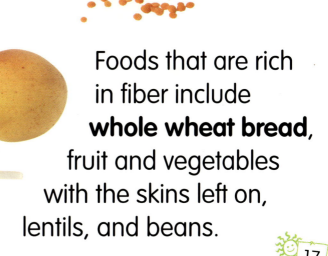

Foods that are rich in fiber include **whole wheat bread**, fruit and vegetables with the skins left on, lentils, and beans.

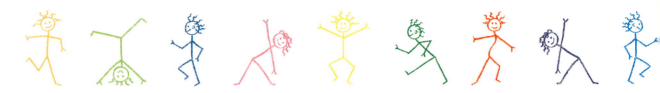

Water for life

You would not live long without water. All the parts of your body need water, so you must have plenty of fluids to stay fit and healthy.

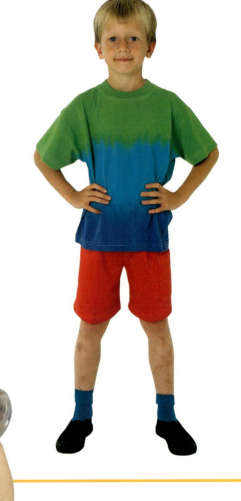

When you are thirsty, your mouth feels dry. This is your body's way of telling you to drink some water.

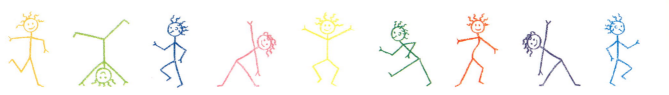

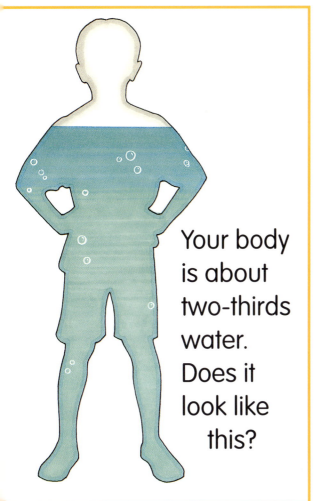

Your body is about two-thirds water. Does it look like this?

You lose water when you **sweat** and when you go to the bathroom. You also lose water when you breathe out.

It's important to replace the water your body loses.

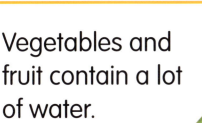

Vegetables and fruit contain a lot of water. Coconut milk is almost all water.

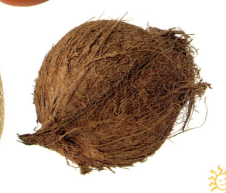

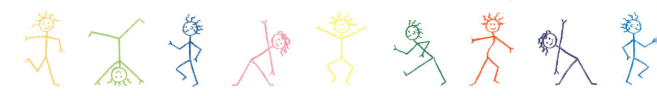

Chewing and swallowing

When you eat, your teeth break the food into tiny pieces. The food is mixed with your **saliva**, and it turns into mushy lumps.

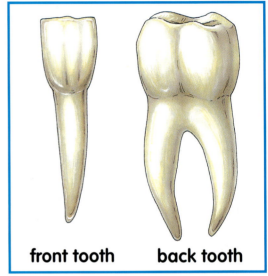

front tooth   back tooth

Your front teeth are used for biting.

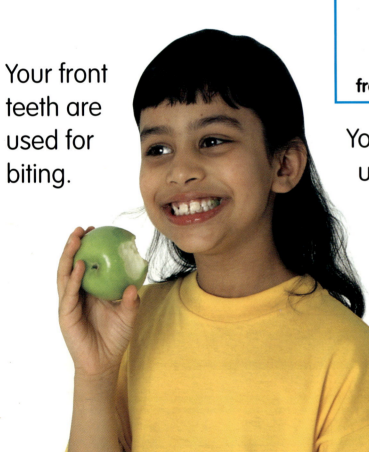

Your back teeth are used for chewing.

Your body breaks down the food and takes the nutrients from it. This is called digestion.

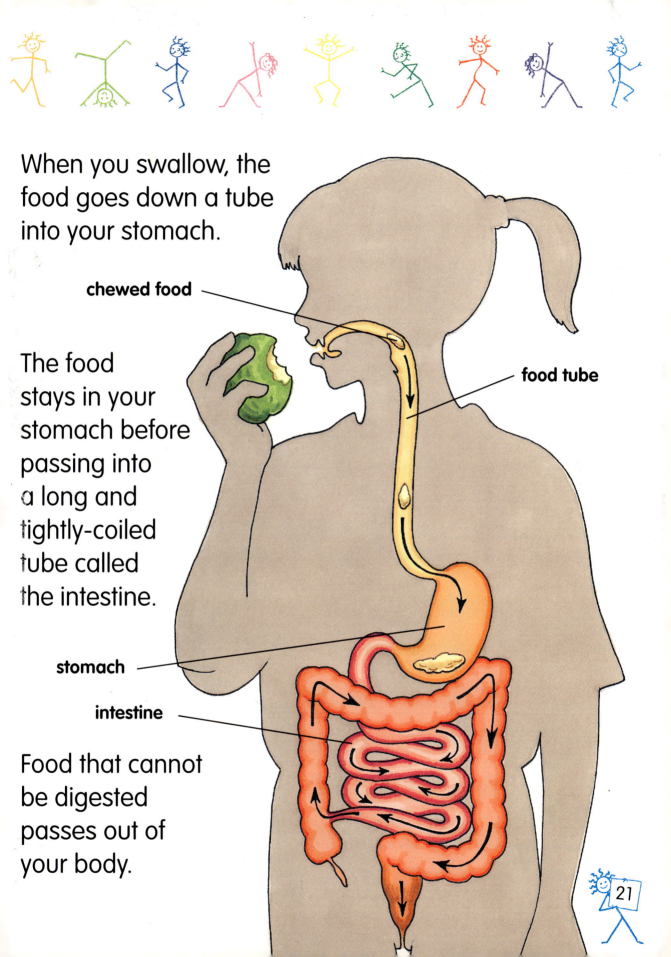

When you swallow, the food goes down a tube into your stomach.

The food stays in your stomach before passing into a long and tightly-coiled tube called the intestine.

Food that cannot be digested passes out of your body.

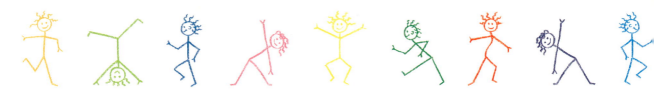

Digesting your food

Inside your stomach, the food is squeezed by your stomach walls and mixed with special **digestive fluids** that contain **acid**, until it is very soft and mushy.

Sometimes your stomach makes funny gurgling noises as your food is being digested.

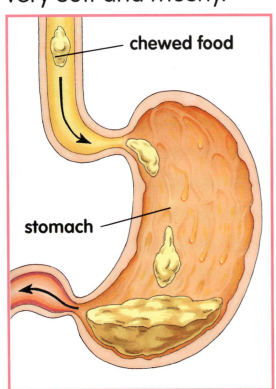

chewed food

stomach

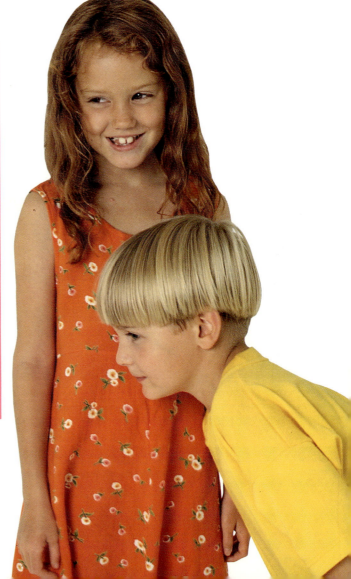

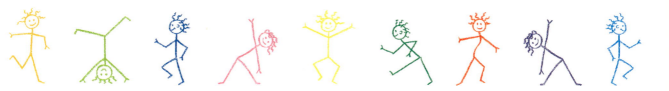

A large meal stays in your stomach for more than three hours. A small meal stays for much less time.

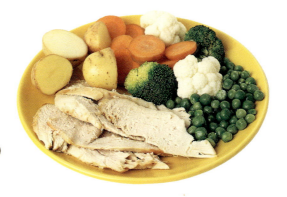

The mushy food passes out of your stomach and into your intestine.

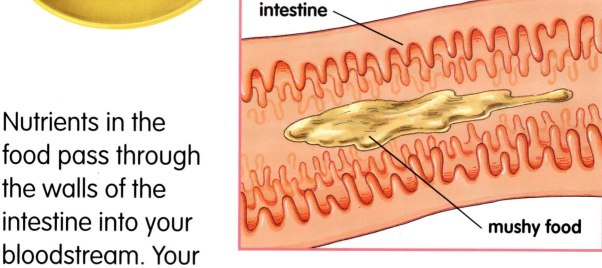

Nutrients in the food pass through the walls of the intestine into your bloodstream. Your **blood** carries the nutrients to every part of your body.

The whole process of digestion takes between 10 and 20 hours.

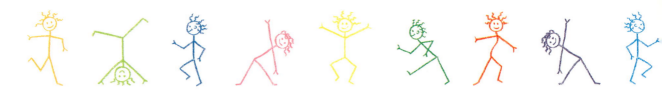

Snacks and junk food

If you ate only chocolate, cookies and potato chips, and only drank soda, you would become unhealthy.

Food that has no nutrients left in it is called junk food. Some **fast foods** are junk food.

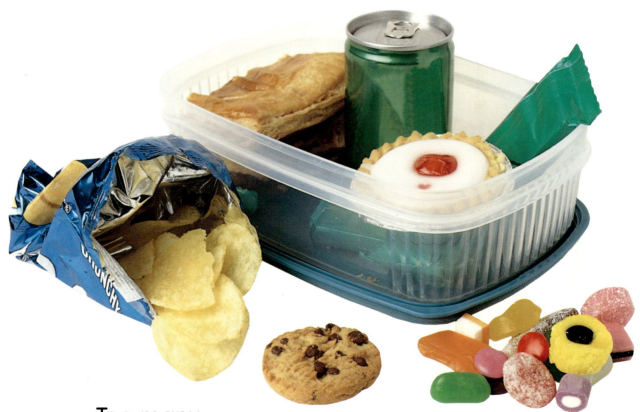

Too many sweet things can make your teeth **decay**.

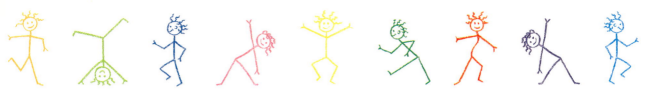

A sandwich made with whole wheat bread, and an apple or pear is a healthy snack for lunch time.

If you feel hungry between meals, eat a piece of fruit or some nuts instead of a chocolate bar.

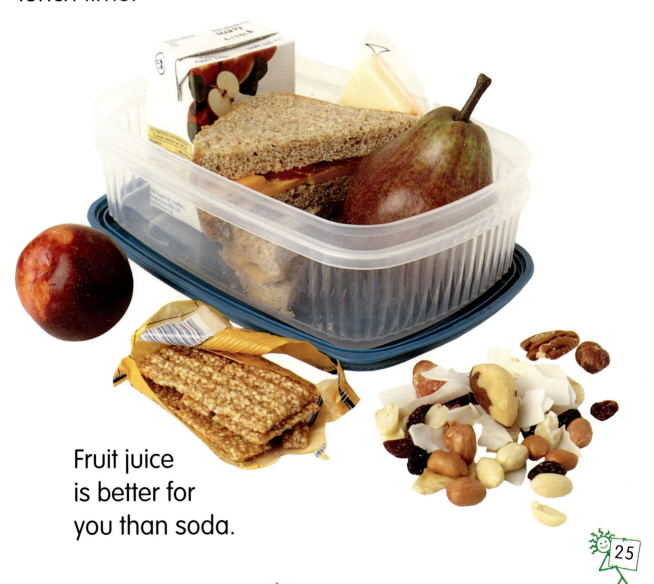

Fruit juice is better for you than soda.

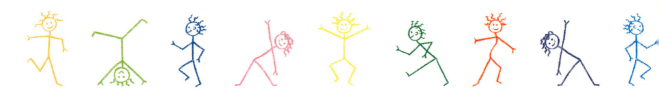

Special food

We need food to live, but we also use it to celebrate birthdays, weddings, and religious festivals.

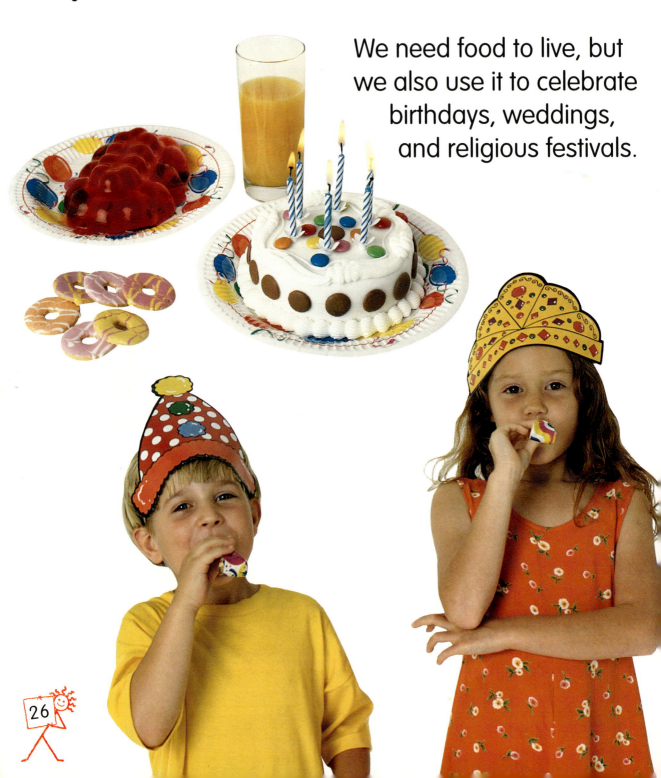

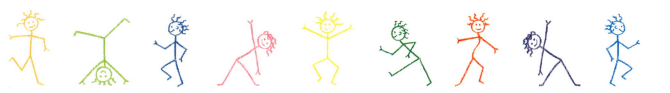

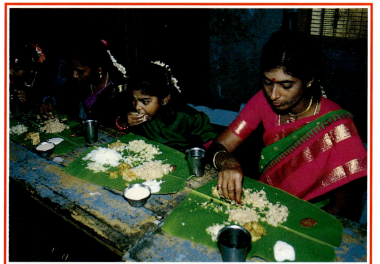

These people are at a Hindu wedding feast. The food has been provided by the bride's family.

Vegetarians are people who do not eat meat. They may believe it is wrong to eat animals.

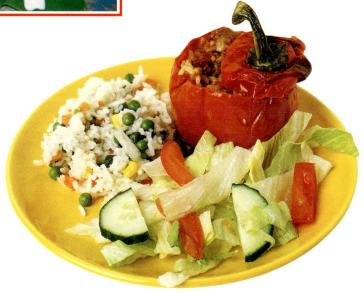

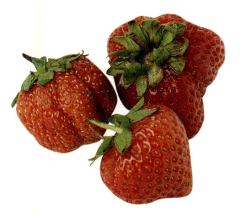

Some people are **allergic** to such foods as strawberries, chocolate, and nuts. If they eat these foods they will become sick.

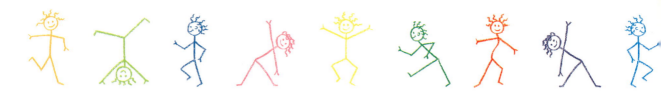

I ate too much!

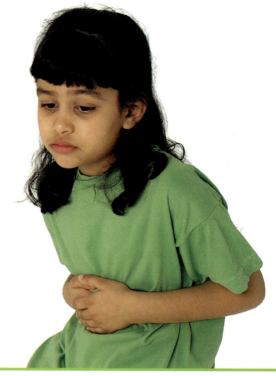

It is not good for you to eat too much of anything at one time. You will get a stomach ache and may even become sick!

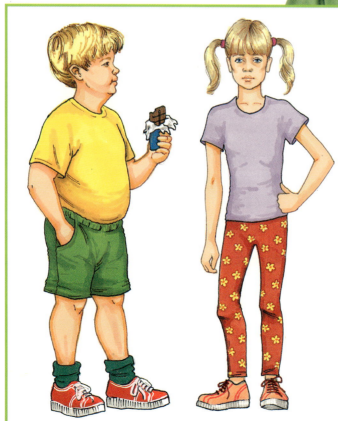

If you eat too much, your body will store the extra food as fat. If you eat too little, you will become thin and weak.

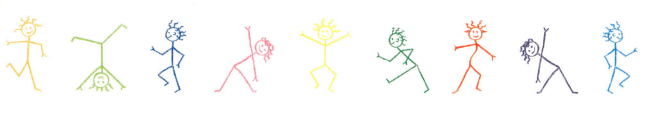

Foods that contain a lot of fat and carbohydrates, like pizza, cake, and burgers, taste nice but don't eat them too often!

You will know if you are eating the right amount for you if you are fit and active, and are neither too thin nor too fat.

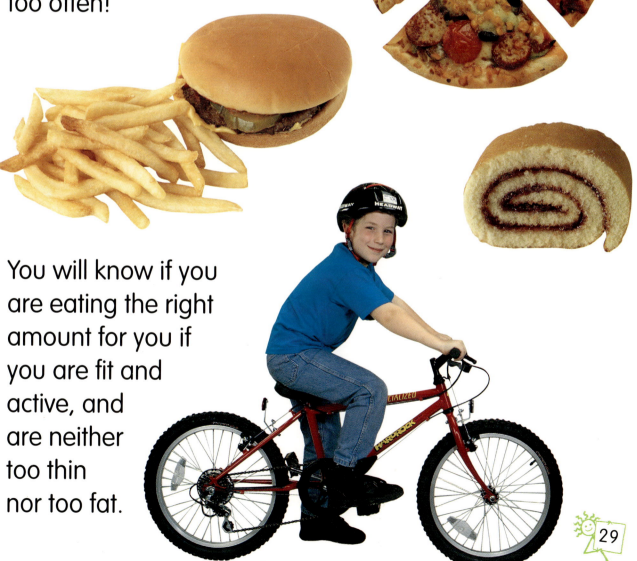

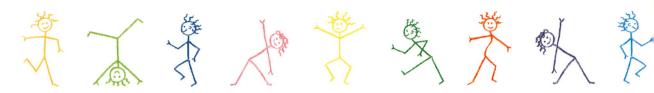

Useful words

Acid
A chemical in your stomach that helps to turn food into a thick liquid.

Allergic
To be sensitive to something. This might be a food which makes you feel ill.

Blood
The red liquid that is pumped around your body by your heart.

Bones
The strong and hard parts inside your body.

Carbohydrates
The part of some foods that give you energy.

Decay
To go bad or to rot.

Digest
To break food up into smaller and smaller parts so that your body can use the nutrients it needs.

Digestive fluids
Liquids in your stomach that help to break down food.

Energy
The ability to play and work without feeling tired.

Fast food
Cooked food that is bought at a quick-serving restaurant.

Healthy
Fit and well.

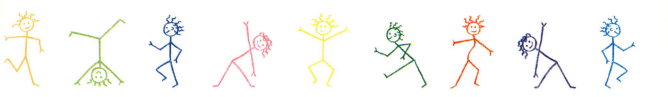

Minerals
Natural substances, such as calcium, that help your body to stay healthy.

Muscles
The soft, stretchy parts inside your body that make your body move.

Nutrients
The useful parts of food that your body needs to stay healthy.

Proteins
The part of food which is used by the body for growth and repair.

Repair
To fix.

Saliva
A liquid in the mouth that prepares food for swallowing.

Samosa
A fried pastry snack filled with meat or vegetables.

Sweat
Moisture from the skin.

Vitamins
Chemicals found in all sorts of food. Your body must have them to help you grow and stay well.

Whole wheat bread
Bread that is made with the whole wheat grain. White bread is made with only part of the grain.

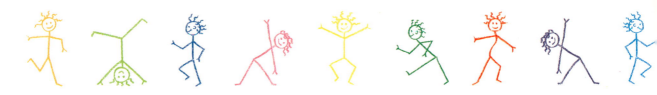

Index

acid 22
allergy 27
avocado 12

beans 9, 17,
blood 23
bones 8
bread 6, 11, 17
burgers 29

cake 11, 29
calcium 15
carbohydrates
 10-11, 29
cheese 6, 9, 12, 15
chocolate 11, 12,
 24, 25, 27
cookies 12, 24

diet 6-7, 13, 16,
digestion 16, 20-21,
 22-23

eggs 9
energy 5, 10, 13

fast food 24

fats 12-13, 29
fiber 16
fish 9, 15
fruit 6, 11, 14, 15, 17,
 19, 25

intestine 21, 23

junk food 24-25

lentils 17

meat 6, 9, 12, 27
milk 9, 13, 15
minerals 14-15
muscles 8

nutrients 4, 6-7, 16,
 20, 23, 24
nuts 9, 25, 27

oranges 15

pasta 11
pizza 29
potatoes 11
potato chips 24
proteins 8-9

religious festivals 26
rice 11

saliva 20
samosas 13
sardines 12
soda 24, 25
stomach 21, 22-23
strawberries 27
swallowing 20-21
sweating 19

teeth 20, 24,
tomatoes 15

vegetables 6, 14,
 15, 17, 19
vegetable oil 12
vegetarians 27
vitamins 14-15

waste food 21
water 18-19
wheat 17
whole wheat
 bread 17